EFFECTIVE APPROACH TO WEIGHT LOSS

AUTHOR: ROBERT JAMES

Terms and Conditions

Table of Contents

Foreword

A multitude of reasons propel individuals who find themselves obese or carrying excess weight to embark on the journey of weight loss. For some, the impetus stems from a deep-seated desire to enhance their overall well-being, striving for a state of health that transcends the mere physical and extends into the realm of vitality. Others are drawn to the prospect of not only feeling better but also experiencing a transformation in their outward appearance, a metamorphosis that has the potential to reshape not only their bodies but also their self-perception and self-esteem.

In a world that demands constant engagement and performance, the aspiration to cultivate higher energy levels becomes a driving force for many. The prospect of having the stamina and vigor to tackle daily tasks with newfound enthusiasm and vigor propels individuals to explore the avenue of weight loss, seeking a revitalization that permeates various facets of their lives.

Yet, irrespective of the unique motivations that propel individuals to embark on this transformative journey, the essence of healthy weight management and the achievement of successful weight loss converge on the foundation of sensibly constructed goals and the cultivation of realistic expectations. It is through the art of setting tangible and achievable objectives that the seeds of accomplishment are sown, allowing for a journey marked not only by milestones but also by the sustainable maintenance of a well-balanced weight.

Chapter 1:

Essentials of Weight Loss Commitment

The idea of losing weight is something many people think about. Some need to do it for medical reasons, while others want to achieve a certain appearance.

Despite the numerous options available in today's market and the easy availability of advice online, reaching your weight loss goals is a different story altogether. People struggle with weight loss mainly because they have incorrect expectations and are misled by the marketing of various products.

Before you rush into starting your weight loss plan, it's important to first consider the fundamental principles of weight loss.

Basics of Weight Loss

Reducing body weight is just one element of a successful and effective weight loss journey. This primary concept is relatable to everyone and can be measured, often yielding visible results. The term "weight loss" encapsulates these ideas.

Weight loss encompasses several crucial factors, including the restoration and enhancement of health, maintaining focus to achieve your weight loss objectives, and transforming and maintaining a leaner physique. To attain successful weight loss, it's essential to adhere to fundamental principles, which consist of the following:

• Shedding fat

• Sustaining motivation

• Building muscle

To achieve success, it's crucial to recognize that shedding those unwanted pounds requires extra effort, as there are no shortcuts in this endeavor.

Lose Fat: Diets Can Help You

Eating a correct and healthy balanced diet is important when losing weight. Choose and follow a diet that is rich in fiber and protein and low in refined carbohydrates.

Once you have increased your intake of fiber and protein, you will lose your weight gradually and your strong muscles will develop. Also, if you consume less refined carbohydrates, you get rid of piling calories, which don't provide the needed nutrients for your body.

Gain Muscles: Do Some Workouts

His path to successful weight loss is not a solitary journey. Sharing your goals, progress, and challenges with someone close can significantly boost your motivation and commitment. Whether it's a friend, family member, or an online support group, having someone to confide in can provide an extra layer of accountability. When faced with tempting treats or unexpected setbacks, knowing that someone is cheering you on can make a world of difference in staying focused and resilient.

Mindful Eating for Long-Term Success

Beyond the realm of exercise, mindful eating emerges as a cornerstone of enduring weight loss success. Gone are the days of eating on autopilot. By engaging in mindful eating, you cultivate a heightened awareness of your food choices and consumption patterns. Savor each bite, appreciating the flavors and textures. Tune into your body's signals of hunger and fullness, allowing these cues to guide your eating. Such an approach empowers you to make conscious and satisfying choices, fostering a healthier relationship with food and preventing overindulgence.

The Role of Rest and Recovery

In the hustle and bustle of life, the value of quality sleep often takes a backseat. Yet, it's a crucial factor in your weight loss journey. Adequate sleep supports your metabolism, helps regulate hunger hormones, and contributes to your overall well-being. Prioritize establishing a consistent sleep schedule and creating a conducive sleep environment. By providing your body with the rest it needs, you're enhancing its ability to recover from workouts, process nutrients efficiently, and optimize your weight loss efforts.

Embracing Consistency and Patience

In a world of quick fixes and instant gratification, it's essential to remember that sustainable weight loss is a gradual process. While rapid changes might lead to initial results, they often prove unsustainable in the long run. Consistency is your greatest ally. Small, steady adjustments to your habits and routines build a foundation for lasting change. Additionally, exercise patience with yourself. Every individual's body responds uniquely to lifestyle changes. Comparing your progress to others' may not accurately reflect your accomplishments. Focus on your journey and the positive steps you're taking each day.

Celebrating Non-Scale Victories

Though the scale's numerical readout can be a measure of progress, there's a world of victories beyond those digits. Celebrate the non-scale triumphs – the increased energy that fuels your day, the improved mood that brightens interactions, and the restful sleep that rejuvenates you. Perhaps it's the satisfaction of comfortably fitting into once snug clothes. These moments, often overlooked, are powerful indicators of your success. Embrace them, for they reinforce the positive impact your efforts are having on your overall well-being.

The Power of Self-Care

Amidst the pursuit of weight loss, self-care is your steadfast companion. Engage in activities that nourish your soul and provide respite from the demands of daily life. Dedicate time to hobbies that ignite your passions. Take moments to relax, whether through meditation, a leisurely walk, or enjoying a good book. By prioritizing self-care, you're reducing stress, enhancing your overall mood, and fortifying your commitment to healthier choices.

Embracing a New Lifestyle

Weight loss transcends numbers on a scale; it's an evolution into a new way of living. Through your journey, you're crafting habits that nourish your body and mind. It's not merely about shedding pounds but about fostering a lifestyle that resonates with your health aspirations. As you integrate positive choices into your daily routine, you're on the path to sustained health and vitality. Each small decision, each mindful choice, propels you toward a life enriched with wellness and well-being.

In weaving these principles into the fabric of your life, you're not just embarking on a temporary endeavor. Instead, you're forging a lasting transformation that honors your body and empowers you with a newfound sense of self. The journey is uniquely yours, and as you embrace these facets, you're stepping into a realm of boundless potential for a healthier, happier you.

Chapter 2:

Integrate Walking

Weight loss is attainable for anyone, contingent on the level of intensity and duration of their walking routine, coupled with their dietary choices. This rationale underlies the advice of numerous experts who encourage individuals dealing with excess weight to incorporate walking as a pivotal aspect of their weight loss endeavor. However, it's vital to recognize that this doesn't imply abandoning a well-rounded, healthy diet. Staying committed to your weight loss strategy remains crucial. Walking serves as an additional element, particularly beneficial for those aiming to witness noticeable results within a shorter span.

Walking As a Bonus to Your Weight Loss Journey

Some people say that physical activities like walking are not important when trying to lose weight. But the truth is, using walks for your weight loss can help you arrive at your desired results.

If you consider adding 30 minutes of brisk walking to your daily activity, you will burn about 150 calories daily. For you to lose a pound every week, you need to get rid of 500 calories each day. Of course, the more you spend your time walking and the quicker your pace is, you will be able to burn more calories.

For you to be successful in losing weight through walking, you need to maintain the intensity of your exercise at a vigorous or moderate level. When it comes to weight loss, the longer you walk or the more intense your walking exercise is, the more calories you'll burn. However, you have to take note that balance is essential.

If you are new to physical activity and regular exercise, you can start at a low intensity and increase it gradually. Once you have succeeded in losing weight, you should not remove your walking exercises from your daily routine as this will help you maintain your weight. Studies showed that people who are maintaining their weight for the long term always consider regular walks. So, keep on walking and ensure to follow a healthy balanced diet.

Guide On How to Use Walking for Your Weight Loss
As previously mentioned, merely engaging in solitary walks won't lead to a successful weight loss journey. It is imperative to also focus on maintaining a nutritious diet to attain your weight loss objectives.

For many individuals striving to shed pounds, adhering to their weight loss plan can prove to be quite challenging. However, this guide aims to inspire and motivate you throughout your weight loss journey.

Monitor Your Dietary Intake

The most effective approach to prevent overconsumption is to vigilantly observe and manage your dietary choices. While it may appear straightforward, overseeing your diet can pose certain difficulties. To safeguard your weight loss aspirations from being compromised, it is advisable to maintain a detailed record of your food and beverage consumption. Additionally, keeping tabs on the calorie content of your meals can be a beneficial practice, enabling you to sustain your desired weight.

1. Measure Your Walks

There are different ways to monitor your walks or how far you have walked. Tracking distance will allow you to compare routes and can assist you in increasing your distance It can also let you burn more calories, which is crucial if you're walking to shed extra pounds.

2 Maintaining a Walking Journal

Keeping a record of your walking activity is just as essential as maintaining a food journal. This practice serves as a valuable tool for staying motivated on your weight loss journey. Moreover, your walking journal enables you to monitor your advancement as you progressively enhance the intensity of your walks.

Chapter 3:
Vitamin-C-Rich Fruits

Recent studies suggest that you can boost your chances of achieving successful weight loss by including more fresh citrus fruits and specific vegetables and fruits abundant in Vitamin C in your diet. While Vitamin C isn't a new miracle cure for weight loss, experts have uncovered that inadequate Vitamin C intake might hinder one's ability to shed pounds effectively.

Getting to Know More about Vitamin C

Vitamin C holds importance beyond its well-known role in cold prevention. In the context of weight loss, this vitamin offers considerable advantages. Surprisingly, fruits abundant in Vitamin C possess the potential to enhance your body's capacity to burn fat. Whether you have weight loss objectives for various reasons, it's noteworthy that this essential nutrient can be a valuable asset in your journey to achieve a healthier weight.

What Is Vitamin C?

Vitamin C, scientifically termed ascorbic acid, falls under the category of water-soluble vitamins and serves a vital role as an antioxidant within the human body. Its primary function revolves around the neutralization of free radicals, which, if left unchecked, can inflict harm upon cellular structures.

Unlike fat-soluble vitamins, water-soluble ones like Vitamin C are not stored within the body's reserves. Consequently, it becomes imperative to consistently introduce fresh supplies of these vitamins into your daily dietary regimen. Failing to do so elevates the risk of developing deficiencies over time, potentially giving rise to a spectrum of health-related issues.

An essential point to note is that the human body lacks the intrinsic ability to synthesize Vitamin C internally. Thus, it underscores the importance of actively incorporating this nutrient into your daily intake, be it through dietary sources or supplementation, to safeguard your overall health and well-being.

Vitamin C and Weight Loss

Incorporating juicing recipes into your weight loss plan can yield favorable results, particularly when you include fruits abundant in Vitamin C.

Currently, researchers are actively exploring fruits and vegetables rich in Vitamin C that have the potential to enhance fat-burning rates during physical exercise. It's advisable to consume these Vitamin C-rich foods and integrate them into your juicing recipes.

While you have the flexibility to choose from a variety of fruits high in Vitamin C, it's understandable if you're unsure about which ones are most suitable for your weight loss journey. In such cases, seeking guidance from experts is a wise approach. Furthermore, if you have allergies to certain fruits, it's prudent to consult your physician for advice on selecting the right fruits that align with your dietary needs and health goals.

Chapter 4:

Exchange Trans Fats for healthier Fat Choices

For a considerable duration, medical professionals and nutrition experts have advocated the benefits of low-fat diets as a primary approach to achieving successful weight loss, averting health complications, and regulating cholesterol levels.

This underscores the significance of understanding the transition from trans fats (considered detrimental fats) to healthier alternatives. The rationale behind this shift lies in the fact that unhealthy fats can elevate your health-related risks, while beneficial fats can serve as protective agents for your overall well-being. It's noteworthy that these healthier fats hold substantial importance not only in the context of physical health but also play a pivotal role in emotional well-being.

Eliminate Trans Fats from Your Diet

Trans fats are normal fat molecules that have been twisted as well as deformed during a process, which is called hydrogenation. In this process, liquid vegetable oil is combined and heated with hydrogen gas. Partially, hydrogenated vegetable oils will make them less likely to spoil and more stable, which is good for all food manufacturers and not a good thing for you especially if you are maintaining a healthy weight.

Trans fats are not healthy. Even a small amount of them is unhealthy. The reason behind this is that these fats contribute to several major health problems like cancer and heart disease.

Fats Sources

When talking about trans fats, many people think of margarine. Well, there are indeed several margarines that are loaded with these fats. However, the main source of trans fats in Western diets comes from snack foods and commercially prepared baked foods.

•   Baked Goods – crackers, cookies, pizza dough, pie crusts, muffins, and other loaves of bread including hamburger buns.

•   Snack Foods – corn, candy, tortilla chips, potato, microwave, or packaged popcorn.

•   Fried Foods – French fries, chicken nuggets, hard taco shells, doughnuts, and fried chicken.

•   Pre-mixed products – pancake mix, chocolate drink mix, and cake mix.

•   Solid Fats – semi-solid vegetable shortening and stick margarine.

Be a Trans Fat Detective

When you go shopping for your weekly or monthly groceries, it's crucial to adopt a habit of carefully inspecting product labels. Always check if any of the ingredients contain trans fats, even if the packaging doesn't explicitly mention them.

When considering margarine for your dietary choices, opt for versions like soft-tub margarine that indicate "zero grams of trans fats." This choice ensures you're avoiding this harmful fat. If you're someone who frequently dines out, it's essential to exercise caution with items like biscuits, certain baked goods, and fried foods. It's advisable to steer clear of these options unless you can verify that the restaurant, you're patronizing doesn't use trans fats in their cooking processes. Additionally, take the initiative to inquire with the restaurant staff about the type of oil they use for cooking. If they mention the use of trans fats, request that they prepare your dishes with olive oil instead.

If you're committed to eliminating trans fats from your diet successfully, one of the key strategies is to reduce or eliminate fast food consumption. It's worth noting that many states lack stringent labeling regulations for fast-food establishments. These foods can be marketed as "cholesterol-free" even when they're cooked in vegetable oil.

How to Choose Healthy Fats

Navigating the array of dietary fats available can indeed be perplexing, but the ultimate goal is to prioritize healthy fats, which offer a wealth of benefits for both weight management and overall well-being.

If you have concerns about heart health or your weight, it's essential to shift your focus away from simply avoiding fat in your diet and instead concentrate on replacing unhealthy fats, such as trans fats, with more nutritious alternatives. This transition may involve substituting some meat with legumes and beans while incorporating olive oil into your cooking.

Here's a breakdown of actionable steps:

Eliminate Trans Fats: When you shop for groceries, always scrutinize product labels to gauge the trans fat content of what you're about to consume. Additionally, reduce your consumption of fast food, as these often contain trans fats.

Limit Saturated Fats: To curtail your intake of saturated fats, consider reducing your consumption of full-fat dairy products and red meat. Opt for healthier alternatives like fish, beans, and nuts, and if possible, include fish in your diet. Furthermore, explore low-fat versions of milk and dairy products as replacements for full-fat options.

Incorporate Omega-3: Make a deliberate effort to include Omega-3 fatty acids in your daily diet. You can source these from foods like walnuts, fish, canola oil, soybean oil, ground flax seeds, and flaxseed oil.

In essence, making informed choices about the types of fats you consume can have a profound impact on both your weight and overall health. Prioritizing good fats while minimizing bad fats can set you on a path toward a healthier lifestyle

How Much Fat is Too Much?

Determining the ideal amount of fat to maintain a healthy weight is a variable that depends on several factors including your weight, age, lifestyle, and overall health status. If you're uncertain about how to gauge your fat intake, it's advisable to seek guidance from experts or establish a personalized fat limit tailored to your specific circumstances. By doing so, you not only set a clear boundary for yourself but also gradually reduce your consumption of unhealthy fats, all while transitioning toward a diet richer in healthier fats.

It's important to note that when embarking on a weight loss journey, it's not just trans fats that should be on your radar as unhealthy fats to avoid. Saturated fats, which are prevalent in various animal-based products, also fall into this category. Lowering your intake of saturated fats can be a pivotal step in effectively achieving your weight loss objectives.

In summary, the amount of fat that is considered excessive for maintaining a healthy weight varies from person to person. Consulting with experts or establishing a personalized fat limit can guide you toward a gradual reduction of unhealthy fats and a transition to a diet emphasizing healthier fats. Additionally, it's crucial to be mindful of both trans fats and saturated fats when striving for weight loss.

Chapter 5

Change Your Mindset Regarding Meal Sizes

In the realm of weight loss, mastering the art of portion control is paramount. Yet, many individuals find it challenging to regulate the sizes of their meals. Initially, this can prove to be a formidable task, but once you've honed this skill, it can revolutionize your approach to eating, allowing you to view portion sizes as a potent tool for both successful weight loss and adopting a healthier diet.

Although meticulously measuring every morsel may not always be practical, it's a valuable starting point to gauge and measure beverages and foods until you develop an intuitive sense of appropriate portion sizes that align with your weight loss objectives.

Surprisingly, even minor distinctions, such as discerning between a single serving and two servings, can wield a significant influence on your progress. Consequently, reshaping your mindset regarding portion sizes becomes a pivotal factor in your weight loss journey, empowering you to make wiser dietary choices and fostering a healthier lifestyle overall.

Understanding Portion Sizes

Commonly, individuals associate serving sizes with the quantities of specific foods they receive when dining out, such as at restaurants. Unfortunately, these portions served are often not in alignment with the true serving size. This discrepancy is a major reason why many struggle with managing their portion sizes effectively.

Even when people are at home, they frequently don't take the time to measure their food accurately. Instead, they rely on estimations to determine what constitutes a single serving of a particular food item. Consequently, this habit can lead to a lack of understanding regarding the concept of true portion size.

To gain a better understanding of portion sizes, it's advisable to actively measure the serving size of your foods. By doing so, you not only gain control over your calorie intake but also acquire the valuable skill of monitoring and adhering to appropriate portion sizes. This practice can be instrumental in promoting healthier eating habits.

People often relate serving sizes to the number of particular foods that are placed on their plates like at restaurants. Unfortunately, that's not what portion sizes are. More often than not, portions that are served are not the true serving size. That is the reason why some find it tough to control portion sizes.

Many people tend to estimate food portions rather than precisely measuring them, even when eating at home. This practice often results in a lack of clarity regarding what constitutes an accurate portion size.

To enhance your understanding of portion sizes, it's recommended that you begin measuring the serving size of your foods. This approach not only enables you to more effectively monitor your calorie intake but also cultivates a better sense of portion control.

Here are some practical guidelines for portion control:

Visualize a serving of fruits and vegetables as approximately the size of a baseball or a closed fist, typically associated with a woman's hand.

Think of a rounded handful as equivalent to roughly half a cup of pasta or cooked rice.

A standard serving size for meat, around three ounces, is roughly comparable to the dimensions of a deck of playing cards.

Picture a large egg or a golf ball to represent about a quarter cup of nuts.

A small potato roughly matches the size of a computer mouse.

While these rules of thumb are helpful, it's important to note that precise measuring remains the most accurate method to ensure you're consuming the right portion size. Initially, measuring can provide you with a solid foundation for portion control. If you're uncertain, consider starting with smaller portions on your plate and, if hunger persists, opt for a second serving. This approach allows you to fine-tune your portion control as you become more attuned to your individual dietary needs.

Chapter 6:

Upgrade Your Mind about Salt and Use Fresh Herbs

Salt itself does not directly cause your body to gain or lose fat, as it contains no calories. However, the consumption of excessive salt can lead to temporary weight gain due to water retention. Conversely, reducing salt intake can result in a temporary loss of weight as your body sheds excess water.

It's intriguing to note that many crash diets promoting rapid weight loss often rely on low or no-salt foods. Nevertheless, this doesn't mean you need to eliminate salt from your diet. You can still use salt if you prefer. However, if you're seeking immediate results and a healthier weight, why not consider using fresh herbs as an alternative to salt? This way, you can not only manage your weight more effectively but also contribute to your overall health and well-being.

Why Change Your Mind about Salt?

Salt is an essential dietary element, but overindulging in it can have adverse effects. Alarming statistics reveal that the majority of Americans exceed recommended salt intake levels. To support your body's proper functioning, a daily consumption of approximately 500 mg of salt is advisable.

What Sodium Does

It's important to note that eliminating salt from your diet is not necessary. Experts advise its use to support essential bodily functions. Sodium, a component of salt, plays a crucial role in maintaining body fluid balance, muscle contraction and relaxation, and the transmission of nerve impulses.

However, an excessive intake of sodium can have adverse effects on the body. It can lead to water retention, increasing blood volume and causing the heart to work harder than usual.

In today's modern food landscape, many products in the market are unhealthy. Therefore, it's essential to make wise choices when selecting foods for your diet, especially if you're aiming for weight loss. Incorporating fresh herbs into your dishes can make a significant difference.

There's a wide variety of fresh herbs available, including parsley, basil, oregano, cumin, thyme, rosemary, chives, black pepper, nutmeg, cinnamon, paprika, and chili powder. These herbs can add savory or spicy flavors to your meals, and some even have a sweet profile. You can pair them with fruits to enhance the taste of healthy desserts and spice up your diet. Fortunately, these herbs are readily available at your local grocery store.

Getting Started When Using Fresh Herbs

For those accustomed to processed and artificial foods, embracing the use of fresh herbs in their meals might appear daunting, especially if it's been a while since they've included such natural ingredients. To make a successful transition to incorporating herbs into your diet, consider the following tips:

Choose Fresh Herbs: The quality of herbs matters significantly. Fresh herbs not only enhance flavor but also offer additional health benefits compared to their dried counterparts. When using fresh herbs, simply chop them finely and follow your cookbook's instructions.

Cultivate Your Herbs: Contrary to the perception of herbs being expensive, growing your own can be a cost-effective and convenient option. Cultivating herbs in your backyard not only saves money but also makes it easier to integrate them into your daily cooking routine.

While adding fresh herbs to your diet is a wise choice, it's prudent to consult with a healthcare professional before doing so. Some individuals may have allergies to specific herbs. To ensure a smooth weight loss journey, identify the herbs that suit you best with the guidance of a medical expert.

Chapter 7:

Alter Your Perspective on Whole Grains

A diet that prioritizes the consumption of whole grains not only helps combat excess belly fat but also lowers the risk of heart disease.

Recent research has demonstrated that individuals who follow weight loss programs incorporating whole-grain loaves of bread and cereals are more likely to achieve their weight loss goals successfully.

Furthermore, those who integrate a diet rich in whole grains experienced a substantial reduction, approximately 38%, in CRP (C-reactive protein), an inflammation marker in the body linked to heart disease.

The research findings strongly indicate that including whole grains in your weight loss journey can contribute to fat burning and a decreased risk of developing heart disease.

Whole Grain Sources

If you're seeking a variety of whole-grain sources to incorporate into your dietary regimen, consider this diverse selection:

- Whole wheat

- Rolled oats

- Popped corn

- Brown rice

- Whole-grain maize

- Entire rye grains

- Millet seeds

- Bulghur wheat

- Triticale grains

- Untamed rice

- Buckwheat groats

- Intact barley grains

- Sorghum kernels

- Quinoa seeds

Moreover, there exist numerous whole-grain alternatives suitable for snacks or meal preparation, including:

- Whole-grain cereal options like toasted oat cereal

- Whole-grain snack crisps

- Utilizing whole-grain flour

- Freshly popped popcorn

These choices offer a wide spectrum of whole grains to enhance the nutritional richness of your diet in various flavorful ways.

If you're seeking a variety of whole-grain sources to incorporate into your dietary regimen, consider this diverse selection:

- Whole wheat
- Rolled oats
- Popped corn
- Brown rice
- Whole-grain maize
- Entire rye grains
- Millet seeds
- Bulghur wheat
- Triticale grains
- Untamed rice
- Buckwheat groats
- Intact barley grains
- Sorghum kernels
- Quinoa seeds

Moreover, there exist numerous whole-grain alternatives suitable for snacks or meal preparation, including:

- Whole-grain cereal options like toasted oat cereal

- Whole-grain snack crisps

- Utilizing whole-grain flour

- Freshly popped popcorn

These choices offer a wide spectrum of whole grains to enhance the nutritional richness of your diet in various flavorful ways.

Whole Grains on the Food Labels

If you are trying to look for foods that contain whole grains, choose foods that have the following:

- Bulgur

- Oatmeal

- Brown rice

- Whole rye

- Whole oats

- Wild rice

- Whole wheat

- Whole-grain corn

If you encounter some labels such as "multi-grain", "bran", "cracked wheat", "seven-grain", or "100% wheat", soon, they don't typically contain whole grains.

You have to take note that color is the basis of whole grains. Some breads can be brown because of their ingredients or molasses. If you want to be sure, check the nutrition facts.

Chapter 8:

Don't Forget the Water

There exist numerous rationales underscoring the significance of water consumption during the process of weight reduction. Hence, it's imperative to keep in mind the necessity of hydrating oneself, as it contributes significantly to attaining your desired weight loss outcomes.

Reasons Why You Should Not Forget Water for Your Weight Loss Resolution

There are various fundamental reasons why incorporating water into your dieting regimen is paramount. This practice is instrumental in averting dehydration, a condition that often accompanies initial weight loss, which is predominantly water loss. It's imperative to ensure proper hydration to counteract this.

Moreover, water plays an integral role in the efficient combustion of fats and calories within your body. Dehydration can hinder this process, slowing down the rate at which your body burns fat and calories. When calories are burnt, toxins are produced, akin to the emissions from a vehicle's exhaust. In this context, water serves as a vital agent for flushing these toxins out of your system.

If your weight loss journey entails sculpting your abs and building muscle, water is indispensable for preserving muscle tone. It aids muscle contraction and acts as a natural joint lubricant, thereby reducing the likelihood of muscle and joint soreness during exercise.

Furthermore, while many recognize the importance of dietary fiber in a healthy weight loss plan, it's essential to understand that without sufficient water intake, you may experience constipation, which can impede your weight loss progress. Therefore, water emerges as a pivotal element in the overall success of your weight loss endeavor.

Chapter 9:

Use Affirmations to Stay on Course

Positive declarations have the potential to set you in motion. This underscores the importance of incorporating affirmations into your daily routine to maintain your trajectory. By understanding the essence of affirmations and their potential influence, you can optimize their effectiveness in your pursuit of weight loss goals.

Affirmations Defined

Affirmations encompass thoughts and expressions, reflecting one's beliefs and expectations in life. These beliefs and thoughts wield considerable influence over the outcomes we experience. For example, if you hold the conviction that weight loss is an insurmountable and formidable challenge, it will indeed manifest as such. Conversely, when you adopt the belief that, while challenging, you possess the capacity to achieve your weight loss objectives, you chart a course toward success. It is crucial to recognize that actions naturally follow thoughts. Therefore, embracing positive affirmations not only nurtures a positive mindset but also propels you toward constructive actions, facilitating your continuous progress.

Navigating the journey toward your weight loss goals poses significant challenges, particularly amid alluring temptations. This is where the practicality of affirmations comes into play. Here are some alternative affirmations to consider:

"I am fully committed to upholding a health-conscious and balanced diet."

"I am dedicated to adhering to a specific dietary plan that amplifies my capability to shed excess weight."

"I am resolute in engaging in one hour of exercise daily, three days each week."

"I am determined to boost my physical activity, such as walking, to enhance calorie burning."

"I am steadfast in following a structured eating routine, encompassing six well-balanced meals throughout the day."

Chapter 10

The Benefits of Maintaining a Healthy Weight

Preserving an optimal weight brings forth a multitude of advantages. It not only elevates the general quality of existence but also extends one's duration of life. Here, we outline the key merits of upholding a healthy weight:

Discomfort Relief

Excess weight can significantly impede one's active lifestyle. Shedding even 5-10% of your body weight can alleviate a myriad of discomforts and aches commonly linked to inactivity.

The additional pounds carried by your body can subject your bones, muscles, and joints to heightened strain, requiring them to exert more effort for even basic movements. Conversely, when your weight is reduced, your body can operate more efficiently and mitigate the risk of injury, thereby facilitating the successful completion of your daily activities.

If your weight is high, your heart might not be able to do its work effectively even if you are resting. However, if you maintain a healthy weight, the amount of blood that is going to various vital organs of the body will increase, which will also allow your heart to do its job efficiently. Maintaining a healthy weight also decreases strains on the heart and reduces one's risk of heart attack, angina, and high blood pressure.

Lower Risk of Diabetes

Based on some research and studies, overweight people are at greater risk of suffering from Diabetes Type II. If you have already been diagnosed with this medical condition, it is important to lose weight as this will allow you to control it in a better way. If you don't have this condition, maintaining a healthy weight will reduce the risks of Diabetes.

Cancer Avoidance

According to various research and studies, individuals who are overweight face an elevated risk of developing Type II Diabetes. For those already diagnosed with this medical condition, effective weight loss can significantly enhance its management. Moreover, for individuals who haven't been diagnosed with Diabetes, maintaining a healthy weight serves as a protective measure, reducing the risk of developing this ailment.

Prevent Osteoarthritis

Osteoarthritis, a condition marked by joint pain, poses a significant risk to many individuals, primarily due to excess body weight. However, maintaining a healthy weight can act as a formidable preventive measure, effectively deterring the onset of this debilitating condition. When coupled with a regimen of regular exercise and a well-balanced diet, the maintenance of a healthy body weight can substantially reduce the strain exerted on your joints. This, in turn, serves as a protective shield, safeguarding your joints from potential long-term damage.

These benefits represent just a glimpse of the myriad advantages associated with sustaining an ideal body weight. If you aspire to lead a healthier life, protect yourself from various diseases, and preserve your physical well-being, embarking on a weight loss journey is undoubtedly a prudent step in the right direction.